Think Eat Move: Weight loss solution

3 Weeks plan with healthy meals recipes

Table of Contents

Introduction...1

My story 4

Part 1: The Metabolism... 6

The Three Basic Rules 13

Part 2: The Road Map Plan... 36

Part 3: Healthy Recipes for Weight Loss..................... 58

First: Healthy Breakfast Recipes 59

Second: Healthy Snack Recipes................................... 68

Third: Healthy Lunch Recipes...................................... 79

Fourth: Healthy Dinner Recipes 92

Conclusion 109

Appendix A...110

Index 114

Introduction

Do you ever wonder why there are so many diets out there and people are still struggling with their weight? Are you curious to know why? I think I know why.

I bet that no matter what you do you still struggling with your weight. You also have a complicated relationship with food (love certain foods and hate another) which impacts your appetite, when you are tired, anxious, or bored you cannot control portion intake even if you are not hungry, this called emotional eating, or a stress-eating. Yet you still have hope that the next diet will stick, or that redoing the diet that worked 5 years ago will work again.

However, it is not going to.

The hardest part is when you find yourself weighing more than you have lost, and when you have a wardrobe full of clothes of all shapes and sizes, that does not fit anymore! And when you get a loser feeling every time you open your wardrobe and keep telling yourself that you haven't tried hard enough, trained enough, or were not motivated enough to follow it. Moreover, this blame will keep you cemented in unnecessary emotional darkness where the only thing that actually helps you feel better is food.

I know all of this very well because I have been their once. After 5 years, with hundreds of books I have read and the people I have met, to end up food addiction, my book is now ready to help you find the best, shortest, easy way in your journey.

In this book, I will help you understand and feel empowered with every change you make.

Now, I want to thank you for choosing this book, 'Think, Eat, Move, a weight loss solution, three weeks weight loss plan with healthy meals recipes', by choosing it, I congratulate you on moving forward to choose a healthy lifestyle.

I will first give out a big secret, this secret is the solution to weight loss and living a healthy lifestyle, it lies in adhering to the three basic rules plan (I personally followed) and stops doing a transient diet, Aligning with Continuity and responsibility is necessary.

This book is written especially for those of you who treat their body as a temple and who are aware and conscious of what choices to make.

We offered many choices in today's world, especially with regard to our food. Some of them are obviously good ones, while others are unhealthy. Whether you choose this book to opt for losing weight or to live a healthy lifestyle using the meal recipes to avoid the temptation of junk food, it will help you. Part 3 included a compilation of some of the most nutritious recipes that are just easy to cook.

There is a popular misconception that healthy food is bland and boring, and through this book, I intend to bust that myth. In this book, you will get access to some of the most delicious breakfast, lunch, snack and dinner recipes, which will help you, lose weight in a healthy manner. All these recipes made from freshly sourced ingredients that are easily available in your local farmers' market. The ingredients are budget-friendly and the recipes are easy to cook, even for a novice cook. By experimenting with these recipes, you will learn that healthy eating can be interesting too and you will completely change your outlook toward your health.

To get the best results with regards to weight loss, I would recommend following this book solution precisely. At the end of the day, it is not just what you eat, but also how you burn it that helps to maintain optimal weight. So what are you waiting for? Let us get started.

My story

My story begins on the day of my son birthday, we were having fun, and he photographed me with his mobile phone and asked me to look at my picture. When I saw it I felt sad, I looked very old, my face is so full and my body gives me more than my real age, and that triggers me, how did I reach this point of weighing 98 kg?

Losing that amount of weight seemed like an impossible challenge, but really, it is not and also it does not mean it is an easy job. Therefore, I started my journey with weight loss through a lot of experiments and errors but ended up succeeding in discovering the best way to lose weight.

Also being an employee was a drain because I was trying to give priority to my health and fitness just as my priority to work. Health must come first, so setting a daily plan of physical activities is essential, and my journey has focused on periods of training, weight lifting and a healthy diet, after all, it became a routine activity in my life.

I lost 25 kilograms, kept it, and I am still losing more only by following the three basic rules included in this book.

Experts always emphasize the importance of adhering to a healthy diet continuously, so far, we do not pay attention to that process.

I found that a secret solution to weight loss lies in adhering to the three basic rules plan and stop doing a transient diet, as well as continuity and responsibility is the secret behind all.

Part 1: The Metabolism

Has it caught your attention that some people maintain their weight stable even if they are eating a huge amount of food? Well, the reason is their metabolic rate, so let us learn about metabolism.

The (Human Body) the calorie-burning machine

The human body is an amazing machine that requires energy to maintain it through complex metabolic processes. However, for many of us, the machine has become slow and ineffective, and partially damaged and rusted.

Anyone who is serious about losing weight and getting a healthy, strong body should first learn how to increase their metabolic rate. In other words, he wants to remove the rust, and launch his own calorie-calorie-burning machine.

What is Metabolism?

Metabolism is one of the vital processes that take place inside the human body. It is responsible for producing energy within the cells of the body by destroying nutrients that digested within the digestive system and converting them to different forms of energy by going through a series of chemical reactions.

Metabolism is the process by which different cells and tissues are constructed and destroyed.

What is the main function of Metabolism?

It is to provide the energy or calories needed to cover body functions or maintain vital functions, thousands of metabolic processes can occur at the same time in the body. One of the most important processes **Muscle metabolism** occurs significantly to maintain, build, and perform the tasks required of it. Therefore, a person with a greater muscle mass does more metabolically than a person with a larger fat mass and has less metabolism.

Metabolism plays an important closely related role in weight loss and weight gain. Those who try to lose weight work to raise their metabolic rate to consume more energy during the day, especially during rest.

A number of factors determine the rate of metabolism in general, such as body size. The more weight and volume of the body, the higher the rate of metabolism, also, the rate of metabolism can be determined by sex, males in general, have a greater metabolic rate than females, and other factors that determine the rate of metabolism is Age.

The magic formula?

A calorie-calorie-burning machine in the body is a simple piece of equipment. In fact, many "experts" make you think that it is more complicated than it is, in order to sell you some products to speed up the process of weight loss. However, all you need to know is some math and some limits in (food, supplements, sports ... etc). Here is the "magic" formula for perpetual weight management.

> Burned Calories - Consumed Calories
> = Net calorie gain or deficit

Do you understand the equation? The calorie intake subtracting the burned calories stored in the sports effort is equal to (=) the net calories stored and consumed.

An accurate estimate of one pound of fat burn is to create a net deficit of 3,500 calories.

Example:

If you burn 500 calories a day more than you consume, you should lose one pound in about 7 days. Conversely, if you take 500 calories a day more than you burn, you will gain a pound in about 7 days.

So here we understand that the basic principle is to have an internal burning food machine for calories in a state of continuous operation at the highest degree.

What do you assume has the greatest impact on your metabolism   (burning more and more calories)?

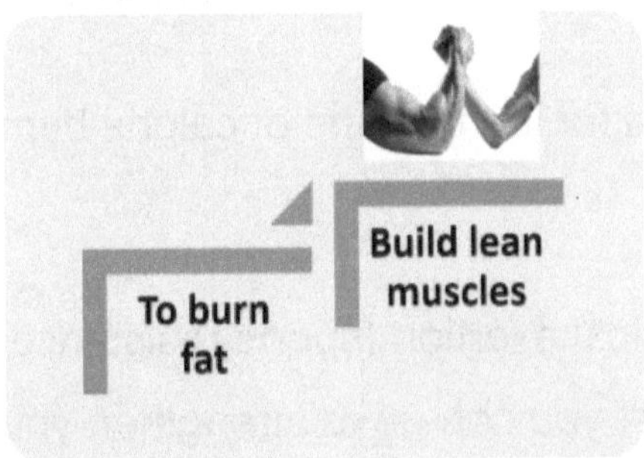

What about the level of activity, thyroid or even age? Maybe heredity, stress or food choices? The answer is none of the above. Although they all affect metabolism (calorie burning), the effect of none of them is comparable to the role of muscle tissue in burning calories. Simply, the more muscular tissue you have, the more calories you burn regardless of other factors. Lean muscle tissue burns calories throughout the day and every day.

Why does Metabolism slow down?

We have all heard that metabolism slows down due to age. Perhaps you have even used it as an excuse for weight gain in the past. However, research has discovered that metabolism DOES NOT slow down significantly due to aging but DOES slow down due to a reduction of muscle tissue.

The main reason for the low rate of calorie burning and muscle loss attributed:

1. Lack of physical exertion (sports resistance exercises, any exercises that you can do to strengthen your body).

2. The general decline in the level of activity with age.

3. Muscle disintegration it usually occurs with a severe diet and skipping meals.

What other factors additional to muscle tissue affect metabolism?

Stress, Meal timing & frequency, Movement level, Food choices, Hydration, Hormones.

The Solution to slow metabolism

1. All you need is an understanding of how your body works

and get a real desire for change.

2. Convert your overall body composition from more fat and less lean muscle to more lean muscle and less fat.

We will determine the approach and the attack plans to follow at the next pages.

The three ideal basic rules to be followed

Continuous calorie burning depends on three important rules that work together in perfect balance. These three rules, if used correctly, lead to a lasting physical and mental transformation.

Many people try to improve their health and transform and slim their bodies using only one or two of these three factors, but it will take them more time to reach the goal they aspire than if they used the three rules if they get there at all.

The three ideal basic rules for continuous calorie burning are:

1. Think.

2. Eat.

3. Move.

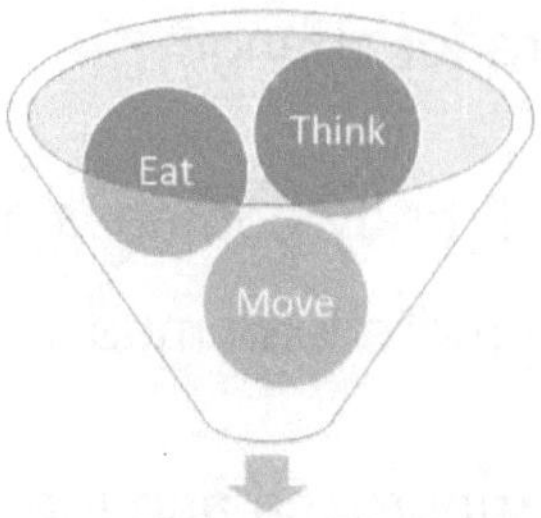

Ideal Inner Food Burning Machine Basic Rules

Throughout this book, we will focus on becoming physically and mentally stronger by learning according to these three factors.

The three ideal rules for continuous calorie burning

Since all three rules that work together on mental and physical transformation will improve your metabolism to burn most calories as quickly as possible, too, you will transform your overall body composition from more fat and less wasted muscles to leaner and stronger muscles.

Whenever you decide to do so without one of the three rules, you actually choose to slow down your metabolism, and thus slow down your physical transformation, it is important to understand that the moment you share all three rules the metabolism (calorie burning) will begin immediate improvement.

The Three Basic Rules

There are two types of Basic Rules in your body: the master rule and the gladiator rules,

Basic Rule 1: Think

It called the Master rule (Mindset and motivation)

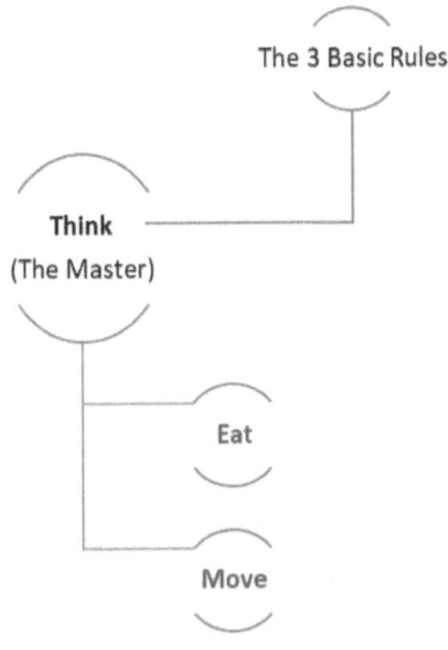

The Gladiators

The master rule transmits power to the two other gladiators so that they can do their work.

The Rule that Master your calorie-burning machine is your mindset, the other two basic rules, which are EAT and MOVE are the gladiators.

We all have our own motives for wanting to make our physical bodies better. For me, my motive was my desire to wear my favorite fashion dresses which I couldn't wear because of my large size (22 UK) and also to choose my clothes from any fashion store which I couldn't do because of my sheer size, believe me, I could only buy from 2 fashion stores

Now, what is your motive? Simply, you want to be stronger and healthier, skinner …etc.

So think about it. What is driving you to make these changes in your life?

Define your goals

As soon as you truly determined your motives behind becoming fit and healthy, the next step is to set a detailed, realistic goal that you simply need to attain over the following three to twelve weeks. Write down your future goals:

- After one month from now

- After 3 month

- After 6 month

- After one year

Doing 'first things first' means Prioritize your life,

In the past, it was difficult for you to start a new exercise routine, monitor your health and dietary habits, but when you put yourself first others will do too.

Believe me, there are other people who may be busier than you are but give their health more time because they know it is vital to accomplish everything else. Prioritization is key. To know that you have chosen your health, take some time to think by writing your goals on paper.

Make the Best Use of Your Time by Scheduling Daily

- It is so important to make a daily plan to achieve your written goals. A daily plan will act as a roadmap to take you to your target.

- Read over your goals daily. If you do not make time for them, you will fall off track.

- You have to set your goals using dates and numbers (ex: I will lose 2 kg by the end of this week)

For me, I achieved the most success when I have successfully learned to engage the three basic rules into my everyday routine. I also found that when I took the time once a week to plan my next seven days, I generate better and faster results.

Therefore, you should do it as I did.

I illustrated an example to be followed later on how to implement the 3-basic rule into your everyday schedule.

Accountability

It is not only your proficiency, but also your accountability, and continuity that determines your success.

What Does Accountability mean?

It means that you are the one responsible for:

- Organizing your time to find space for planning,

- Measuring your progress,

- Writing your goals every single day, and place them on your calendar or fridge to check them to know which is achieved.

- The fact that sometimes we need support for encouragement to stick our goals. I encourage you to have a personal trainer (if you can afford it) or a friend, husband, or a family member to support you in your journey to becoming the person you desire.

The daily planning process will help you visually analyze your daily achievements and create a stronger consciousness of the new habits that you are forming.

Another powerful tool that will help you in your transformational experience is writing down your thoughts, feelings, and experiences in a notebook, or record success on video.

Basic Rule 2: Eat

Between 70 and 80 % of the way you look and feel **depends** on what you put in your mouth. No single factor can equal the effect of nutrition on your body's transfer of fat to lean muscles and improve metabolism.

Regardless of your age, level of physical activity, taking or not taking supplements, if nutrition is weak and incorrect, it is almost impossible to achieve good overall health and wellness. Nutrition is certainly the first factor to be addressed in order to change your health and fitness it will provide your body with the tools it needs to transform your shape forever.

Focus on nutrition first and you will start to see results faster with less effort.

Guidelines to Nutrition

I have tried all kind of diets, new and old fashioned not only to get the transformation that I need; but also to make it last, and at the same time live my life happy and not feeling angry because of missing the passion of food , I found that the best effective way to nutrition is to follow these guidelines:

1. Eat at predetermined close times.

2. Eat the right types and proportions of foods

3. Eat the Correct Portions and Combinations.

a. Must read labels of packaged food

4. Prepare Your Food in Advance.

5. Drink water.

Guideline 1: Eat at predetermined close times

You should eat every 2-3 hours, 5-7 times a day. Determining the best times to eat depends on when you wake up, when you exercise and when you go to sleep.

I suggest that:

- Eat your first meal within an hour of waking up; your body's (burning rate) is high and needs fuel to keep your fat-burning going.

- Eat 30 minutes before exercise. This gives you a boost of energy to work out, which in turn burns more calories,

Guideline 2: Eat the right types and proportions of foods

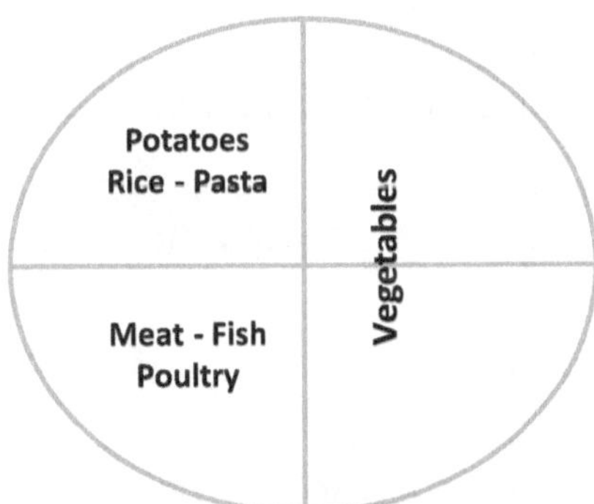

Your plate should contain :

Choosing the right types of foods is not as complicated as some hold.

The food you should avoid: pizza, fast food, sweets, candy bars, chips, and processed foods.

Here is a quick analysis of the best foods and their benefits:

Proteins and their benefits

It is important to eat protein at every meal when you consume a carbohydrate

The primary role of Protein is:

- Build and repair tissue

- Plays a major role for almost all enzymes.

- It helps you to be more satisfied for a longer period.

- It helps you eat less carbohydrate

Check the following:

Eggs are the perfect food to eat because our bodies use all protein in them, also grass-fed beef is healthier than corn-fed beef.

Carbohydrates and their benefits

1. Carbohydrates ("carbs") function primarily as an energy source.

Carbs are contained of simple carbs and complex carbs, Once consumed, your body converts both types of carbs to glucose for energy,

a. Simple carbs:

i. Table sugar, sugary drinks, candy, cake, baked food from white flour, fruit juice.

ii. Tend to spike blood sugar levels, giving a quick energy boost, often followed by a crash as the rest of the energy is converted to fat, resulting in moodiness, reduced energy, and cravings for more sugar

b. Complex carbs:

i. Whole grains, brown rice, and most vegetables.

ii. More difficult for the body to convert this type to glucose, and the digestion process takes longer, are naturally low on the glycemic

Check the following:

Aim to eat organic or local or farm-fresh food as possible and include different colors of vegetables every day. Avoid sugar and dairy, which not labeled organic. When looking at a canned food recipe, a protein bar or a frozen meal pay attention to:

- Sugar must be less than 7g.

- It should not include high fructose sugar, modified cornstarch, refined flour.

Fats and their benefits

Fat is a strong and intense source of energy, its crucial for a healthy immune system and has a greater benefit for the heart and brain.

There are two types of fats:

- Unnatural fats (saturated and trans fats).

- Natural fats (monounsaturated and polyunsaturated) like olive oil, avocados, nuts, and seeds are a great addition to every meal.

- Try to include 20-30% of fat daily. (ex. equal to 40-60 grams for a 2000 calorie diet).

Fatty acids (fish oil, flaxseed oil, hemp seed oil, and Grapeseed oil) help us to increase our metabolism rate. Also, help to enhance memory concentration, slowing the aging process (skin, hair, and nails),

Check the following:

- Do not heat oils to smoking levels.

- When looking at a canned food recipe, a protein bar, or a frozen meal: do not choose the ones written on it (NO Trans fatty acids), or the once contains hydrogenated soybean oil.

- Coconut oil and Coconut milk are healthy fats it is good for you.

Guideline 3: Eat the Correct Portions and Combinations

In my 4-year experience, I have determined that a good combination is to make sure that each meal combined of (45-55%) carbs, (30-45%) protein, and (20-30%) as fats.

This combination provides the body with the required protein, fats and energy.

Check the following:

When looking at a canned food recipe, a protein bar, or a frozen meal: Protein in grams is half or more of the carbohydrates in grams to be a complete meal, The sodium is less than 500mg.

Guideline 4: Prepare Your Food in Advance

Once it is done right, meal preparation will help you stay motivated, scheduled and, most of all, prepared for any scenario, remember that busy world we all live in,

That is exactly why if you do not prepare your meals in advance, you are asking for failure.

You must:

1. Plan your week menu in advanced

2. Go shopping for the whole week meals menu (organic or local grocery), if you use any canned products wash them with excess water before use

3. Make one day for cooking, it's better to be in your weekend

4. Try to make meals from basic ingredients

5. Make multiple batches of the same meal

6. Around two days meals put in the fridge, the rest store in the freezer

7. Each meal should be combined of (45-55%) carbs, (30-45%) protein, and (20-30%) as fats.

These steps are simple but must be followed for an optimal

outcome. Nutrition is what will make the difference.

Guideline 5: Adequate body hydration (Water intake)

Water will actually help get rid of body fat and in muscle recovery, so it is important to get the right amount.

1. Drink 3-4 liters of water per day (12-16 8 oz. glasses of water)

2. Carry a reusable water bottle wherever you go.

3. Drink the majority of your water prior to 5-6 p.m. This can help with water retention

How to drink and when to drink it really has a lot to do with your activity level, health conditions and if you are on any medications that may make it dangerous to drink this suggested amount. If drinking this much water is simply overwhelming, then take it one glass at a time, and try to add one more glass every other day. You will be surprised how much this will affect your weight loss and energy levels.

Here are some benefits of drinking water:

1. To help the liver and kidney to break down fat or converting stored fat into energy.

2. Water intake control and decrease your cravings

3. It is the main transporter of food and waste,

4. It's will increase your skin tightness, resulting in a much younger look.

Supplement for more enhancement

To enhance your results, take:

- **Multi-Vitamins**:

- Supports overall health and immune system

- I recommend using a multi-vitamin created from whole foods. I believe this is the best kind to take because whole foods break down naturally, it can be taken on an empty stomach, and do not give you a nauseated feeling.

- **Crucial Fatty Acids**

- I mean the omega fats. Fatty Acids are important for a fitness-oriented lifestyle and overall health. Also, it assists in energy production, diffusion of oxygen into the bloodstream, and brain.

- They help in strengthening the immune system, reduce water retention by removing sodium and water, and help in mood regulation.

- They help to increase skin tone and enhance your vision

- **Supplements for muscles recovery:**

a. A recovery supplement aids in the rebuilding of the muscle, allowing it to rebuild quicker so that you feel stronger and healthier.

b. L-Glutamine is an amino acid used to elevate the immune system, also allows your muscles to use the protein for growth.

c. You should take a recovery supplement directly after your workout and right before bed.

- **Thermogenic (Curbs appetite and boosts energy)**

- Thermogenic supplements support weight loss through increased body temperature, which increases metabolism, energy levels, which leads to burning more calories.

- They also reduce appetite.

- Research studies have determined that thermogenic a powerful effect on weight loss, burning fat and reducing water content in the body.

Examples of popular thermogenic:

- Garcinia Cambodia, Green Tea, cayenne, chili pepper,

ginger.

- Lime with water drink.

- Cucumber, mint, and lime mixed in water,

- Matcha green tea powder

- **Whey Protein (Promotes muscular development)**

The Whey protein should contain (zero fat, zero carbs, and zero sugar, around 25-gram protein). Reasons why we should include whey protein as part of our healthy life:

- Whey Protein is an immediate muscle supply.

- Regular to small amounts of protein balance blood sugar to reduce pains, muscle weakness, and dizziness.

Optimal times for best results:

- First thing in the morning

- Last thing before going to bed

- Right away before and after work out.

Basic Rule 3: Move

Remember, the goal of turning yourself into a calorie-burning machine is to transition your body mass from fat to lean - muscle tissue. Let me tell you some facts about building muscle tissue by moving.

Moving is equal to Strength Training and cardio training this perfect combination completes each other, the first to build muscles the second to burn fat.

Do not choose between them, do both of them

Move =: Strength Training + cardio training

Benefits with Strength Training:

- Will build Muscular tissue and lean body mass throughout regular resistance training. If your aerobic workout not balanced with an appropriate strength training system, you lack an important component of overall health and fitness.

  "You will never get bulky if you lift weights."

- Strength training is the best way to lose body fat and have a new body, looks tighter skinner with muscles.

  "The more muscle you have, the more calories you burn."

- It will build back the lost muscle tissue that usually occurs with aging.

- It will control your weight by increasing metabolism, and gaining muscle,

- It will reduce the risk of injury, and improve your focus

Benefits with Cardio Training:

If you add cardio training immediately following your resistance session, this will give you a big metabolic boost. Therefore, if you perform the two back-to-back, you enhance the metabolic function of your body and reap additional rewards in the form of fat loss and muscle gain.

Cardio training to follow for the next 3 weeks:

o 20-45 minutes/day 4-6 days/week.

o Day 6 is always an optional cardio day, either to work out for this extra day to lose more or enjoy the day off.

o You should be breathing hard that you could barely inhale and exhale from your nose.

If you have any health condition, you may want to consider doing a Moderate exercise instead which can help your situation: such as only (walking or cycling) for 45 minutes a day.

Benefits of Rest for recovery.

- Getting enough sleep for 8 hours every night. In addition, your sleep should begin at 11: 00 p.m.

- For the next 3 weeks, resolve to be asleep by 11: 00 p.m., which means you have to be in bed earlier.

- The correct amount of rest will Improve muscle recovery, and reduces water retention.

Before Starting Transformation

Before we start working together, I share two main things with you so that we are all on the same page of this process:

1. Commit to getting out of the malnutrition that you are in

2. Commit to renewing your goals and subconscious habits

Most diets fail because they focus mostly on logical and sometimes on physical parts to help someone lose weight, But they neglect the main reason why people who start a diet return to their old habits within a period of time.

They forget the state of mindset, which consists of setting goals and resetting the subconscious mind.

This subconscious is those habits you do not think of. Once you do something often, your mind puts it on autopilot and saves space in the logical brain for something else. They are in autopilot because you have been doing them for so long. Like the way you brush your teeth, how you fold the laundry, the same thing applies to the way you eat.

Therefore, in your past years, you have built some unconscious routine in your mind about food, now you have to reset them with new ones be about food is that the missing puzzle you have been looking for a long time.

We can't dive directly into the subconscious mind from day one, because mind don't make this change only after 3 to 12 weeks and it will be gone forever, it's hard to renew the habits that were with you As long as you can remember them.

But the most important part of the success of all of this, its **commitment.**

Commitment to work.

Commit to going out a little out of your comfort zone.

Commit to appearing, opening up, and having fun in the process.

I think you have this level of commitment here because you read these lines, so, if you feel this book is talking to you, welcome to an amazing journey together that will help you achieve your goals!

So, without further waiting, let us start!

Transformation

No matter what fitness goals you have set, you can bet that your body will experience changes as you follow a healthy lifestyle. Everyone reacts differently to changes in nutrition and exercise, but you can expect a range of changes along the way.

Before we start working together, I share two main things with you so that we are all on the same page of this process:

3. Commit to getting out of the malnutrition that you are in

4. Commit to renewing your goals and subconscious habits

Weeks 1-3: Create New Habits

- You will form new habits

- Many people experience a great weight loss within the first few weeks of starting the program.

Weeks 4-6: Look and feel smaller

- You will begin to realize that your clothes are being lost and you will look and feel thinner in the face and neck.

- In addition, you will have greater levels of energy.

Weeks after: More Achievements, and Higher Ability

- You will notice that excess fat has melted away.

- New habits are now a healthy lifestyle. Your old body transformed into the one you desired.

- Now you have the perfect knowledge to eat smart and exercise effectively

Part 2: The Road Map Plan

BURNING CALORIES

THE PLAN TO FOLLOW

Now that you become educated with the three basic rules, it is time to start! Review the guidelines below to ensure your success.

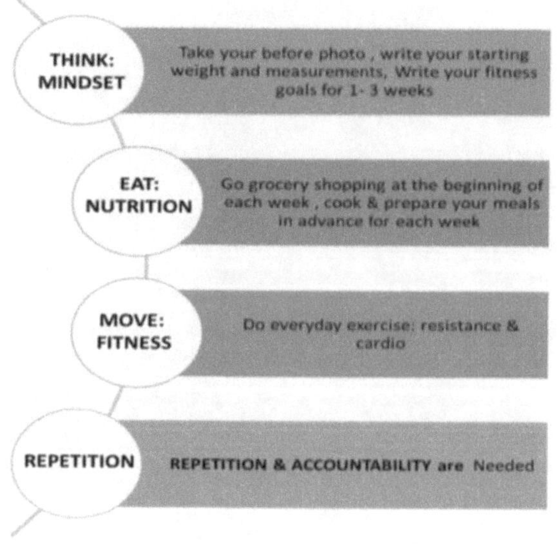

Take the before transformation photo

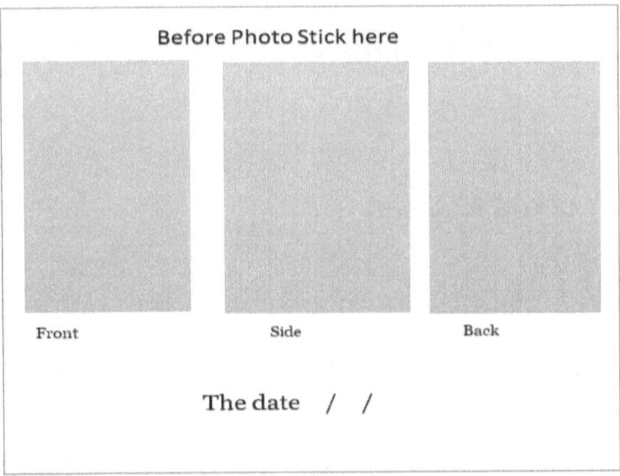

(Hint: a photo taken at the same distance, angle and lighting, wear tightfitting clothing to permanently reveal actual changes, keep the tightfitting cloth for more pictures)

Write several sentences to explain the states of your mood:

Writing motives & goals strategy

Time to get to work.

- Make a list of motives and goals as well as the changes you would like to see in your body (be specific). Knowing your motivation is a key characteristic behind successful goal completion.

- Make your goals realistic.

- Make your goals measurable, is important because you can compare how much you achieve in every level

- Make your goals small (set attainable goals) to keep yourself motivated

- Keep your goals in sight, where you can see them on a daily basis to set focused and inspired.

- Read your Affirmation Statements & motivations, and goals every morning

Identify your motives and goals by answering these questions (process goals):

What is driving you to make these changes in your life? (Physical and emotional) dig deeper and make it real.

Are you losing your weight for yourself or for someone else?

The main motive: --

The minor motives: ---

By the end of the next 3 weeks: what results do you want to see?

Weight? Measurements? Body shape?

What are the benefits of achieving your goals? State your reasons and desire to change your lifestyle?-----------------------

----

List all of your friends, family members & resources that will support you to achieve your goal.

Indicate the difficulties that can prevent you from achieving your goal (time, responsibility, money, etc.)

What behavior you should adopt to succeed with your goal? (
wakeup early, sleep early,

Make a plan:

Describe your plan of action in detail:

3 weeks plan

Sleeping and waking up times --

----

period between meals --

---grocery shopping days:

---meals you are going to eat
(choose from the recipes, the same 3 meals for each week, if
you don't like and have the time to cook choose more meals)

Week1: ---

--------------------week2: --

------------------------------------week3: ------------------------------------

----

You can use the daily plan schedule in the following pages for an everyday plan.

Do the same for:

 12 weeks plan

----

24 weeks plan

A Daily Plan schedules

	As soon as you wake up, THINK: Review and re-commit to your goals
7:00 AM	EAT: Eat a meal, Take Supplements, Drink water
8:00 AM	
9:00 AM	Drink Whey Protein, MOVE: Resistance training, Cardio training, Drink water
10:00 AM	Take your thermogenic supplement (Garcinia Cambodia, Green Tea or ....)
11:00 AM	EAT: Eat a snack, Drink water
12: 00 AM	
1:00 PM	
2: 00 PM	EAT: Eat a meal, Drink water (20-30 mins)
3:00 PM	
4:00 PM	EAT: Eat a snack, Drink water
5:00 PM	

6:00 PM	
7:00 PM	EAT: Eat a meal, Drink water
8:00 PM	
9:00 PM	EAT: Eat a snack **or** drink whey protein, Take Supplements, Drink water
	Plan for tomorrow, Drink water, sleep 8 hours for muscles recovery
*Make your daily plan based on your life, the time you wake up and the time you sleep	

Tracking weight loss progress schedule

	DATE	BUST	WAIST	HIP	Arm Circumference
BEFORE STARTING					
CHANGES					
WEEK1					
CHANGES					
WEEK2					
CHANGES					
WEEK3					
CHANGES					
WEEK4					
CHANGES					
WEEK5					
CHANGES					
WEEK6					

CHANGES					
WEEK7					
CHANGES					
WEEK8					
CHANGES					
WEEK9					
CHANGES					
WEEK10					
CHANGES					
WEEK11					
CHANGES					
WEEK12					

* Arm Circumference: This is a measurement around the fullest part of your upper arm.

Nutrition strategy

The following pages walk you through the Nutrition Strategy. As you follow the daily nutrition plans, remember to refer back to this section to keep you on track.

- Eat your meals on schedule:

o Eating every 2-3 hours will keep your metabolism constantly burning.

o Eat your morning meals every 2 hours and afternoon meals every 2.5-3 hours.

o Eat your first meal within the first hour of waking in the morning.

- Eat the same meals only for one week

o For each meal, eat the same thing every day for one week; By eating the same meals daily, your metabolic burn will increase.

o By always knowing what and when to eat, you will find building new lasting habits much easier.

- Follow the meal plan strictly unless you feel you are eating too much or too little, have an allergy to specific foods.

- Do not snack a lot: By snacking, you lose track of calorie count, strictly avoid taking "just a bite" of this or that of something not on the plan.

- Protein is important, it has to be included before and after the workout

Nutrition intake timing as in Daily Plan schedules

- Breakfast

- Energy snack

- Lunch

- Energy snack

- Dinner

   Do not forget to include in your schedule:

   - Pre-workout **whey** protein

   - **Whey** protein before sleep

   - Thermogenic supplements

   - Water

* Nutrition recipes added later in the book

Meal preparation

- Make your first week plan by choosing your meals from the meals I included later in this book.

- Go shopping and get all the food on the shopping list you made from the recipes you already choose

- Prepare a big amount of meals: Measure your exact portions. Cook for the week

- Chop the fresh vegetables and fruits to put them in separate containers for either each day or all in one container that you measure out each day.

- Assemble meals: either each meal separately (in containers, bags, etc.) or keep all the food in bulk and measure out each time they prepare their food for the day.

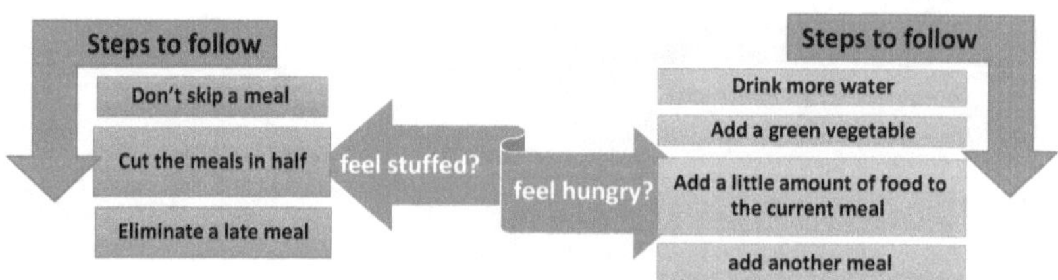

- If you feel stuffed:

o If you are feeling stuffed, the most important thing to know is to NOT skip any meal

o Keep eating on your scheduled times; do not go more than 3 hours without eating.

o Cut the meals in half: Whatever meal is making you feel stuffed cut both your protein AND your carbs in half. Do not only cut a carb or only a protein; make sure to cut the entire meal in half.

o If cutting a meal in half just is not doing it and you absolutely have to cut a meal out, choose to cut Meal 4, 5, or 6. But only cut out one meal at most

- If hungry:

o Congratulations! If you are starving, this is a **positive indication that your metabolism has increased**

- Drink more water

- Add a green vegetable

- Add a little amount of food to the current meal when you happen to be hungry.

- If none of the above are doing the trick, it is time to add another meal. Stack the first four meals every 2 hours and the last three meals every 2.5-3 hours.

Fitness method

The fitness method: six days of workouts per week. Three of the days, you will do your cardio training with your resistance training. Ideally, you should do the resistance training and cardio sessions back-to-back, starting with resistance training. Your cardio workouts on non-lifting days will be more intense, in the form of interval training.

Two examples A and B workout to follow:

Important: If you have any health condition, you may want to consider doing a Moderate exercise instead which can help your situation: such as only (walking or cycling) for 45 minutes a day.

Workout A: in a lifting day

push	pull	legs	core
Push up	Lat-pull Down	Single leg press	Prone cobra
Standing dumbbell press	Rear lateral raise	Lying leg curl	Woodchop
Seated chest press	Seated row	Body squat	Reverse sit up

Dumbbell lateral raise	Bent row	Hip bridges	Plank
Cardio		-------	30-40 minutes
Perform each exercise for 30-45 seconds to start, then increase the duration			

Workout B: in a lifting day

Incline chest press	Seated high row	Dumbbell squad	Dead bug
Flat dumbbell press	Single-arm row	Back lunge	Plank
Single-arm dumbbell press	Banded rear raise	Romanian deadlift	Seated twist
Standing barbell press	Assisted pullup	Seated leg curl	Hyperextension
Cardio		-------	30-40 minutes
Perform each exercise for 30-45 seconds to start, increase the duration			

Cardio workout: in a NON-Lifting day

Walking or running	intensity	duration	sets
WARM-UP		10 min	1
	high	1 min	10

	low	1 min	10
Cooldown		5 min	1
	total	35 min	22

**Total workout time: Max Muscle's workouts will take roughly 45 minutes. As you, get more familiar with the program

Part 3: Healthy Recipes for Weight Loss

Everyday Snacks, Breakfast, Lunch & Dinners

First: Healthy Breakfast Recipes

Quinoa Breakfast Bake

Serves: 4-5

Ingredients:

- ¼ cup quinoa, rinsed, drained
- 1 ½ medium, very ripe bananas, peeled, sliced
- ¼ cup raspberries
- ¾ cup blueberries, divided
- ¼ cup steel cut oats, uncooked, rinsed, drained
- 2 tablespoons coconut flakes, unsweetened, toasted (optional)
- 1 large egg or ¼ cup egg whites or ¼ cup flax eggs
- 1-1 ½ tablespoons maple syrup (optional)
- ½ teaspoon pure vanilla extract
- A pinch salt
- ½ scoop protein powder (optional)
- ¼ teaspoon ground cinnamon
- 1 cup milk of your choice

- Cooking spray

- Yogurt to serve (optional)

Directions:

1. Add eggs, milk, protein powder, maple syrup, salt, cinnamon, and vanilla extract into a bowl. Whisk well.

2. Grease a baking dish (7-8 inches) with cooking spray. Spread half the blueberries, bananas and raspberries in the dish.

3. Spread the quinoa over the fruits. Next layer with steel-cut oats.

4. Place the remaining blueberries, bananas, and raspberries on top.

5. Gently pour the egg mixture at the corners of the dish and not directly in the center of the dish. This is to prevent the fruits from floating to the top.

6. Sprinkle toasted coconut flakes.

7. Bake in a preheated oven at 375 ° F for around 45-60 minutes.

8. Remove from the oven and cool for a while. Cut into 4-5 equal slices.

9. Serve hot or cold or warm, topped with yogurt if using.

Chia Seed Omelet

Serves: 1

Ingredients:

- 2 eggs

- 1 teaspoon chia seeds

- ½ chopped cup tomatoes

- 1 teaspoon olive oil

- 1 cup baby spinach

- Salt to taste

- Pepper to taste

Directions:

1. Add eggs into a bowl and whisk well. Add salt and pepper and beat again.

2. Place a small nonstick pan over medium heat. Add oil. When the oil is heated, add spinach, chia seeds, and tomatoes and sauté for a couple of minutes.

3. Pour egg on top and swirl the pan so that the egg spreads.

4. Cook until the eggs are set to the desired doneness. Gently slide the omelet onto a plate and serve with toast.

Oatmeal Cinnamon Raisin Smoothie

Serves: 2

Ingredients:

- 2 cups soymilk

- 6 tablespoons old-fashioned oats

- 1 ½ teaspoon ground cinnamon

- 2 scoops protein powder

- 2 large overripe banana sliced, frozen

- 4 tablespoons raisins

- ½ teaspoon vanilla extract

Directions:

1. Add all the ingredients into a blender and blend until smooth.

2. Pour into two glasses and serve.

Honey-Lemon Ricotta Breakfast Toast with Figs and Pistachios

Serves: 4

Ingredients:

- 4 slices whole-grain or gluten-free bread

- Juice of a lemon

- 8 figs, sliced

- 2 teaspoons lemon zest, grated

- ½ cup low-fat ricotta

- 1 tablespoon honey

- 4 tablespoons pistachio, chopped

Directions:

1. Toast the bread slices to the desired doneness.

2. Meanwhile, add ricotta, honey and lemon juice into a mixing bowl.

3. Whip until creamy.

4. Spread this mixture over the bread slices. Place fig slices on top. Garnish with pistachio and lemon zest and serve.

Avocado Toast and Egg

Serves: 2

Ingredients:

- 4 eggs

- 2 small avocadoes, peeled, pitted, mashed

- 4 slices multi-grain or whole wheat bread

- Salt to taste

- Pepper to taste

- 2 teaspoons lime juice

- A handful of fresh parsley leaves, chopped

Directions:

1. Add avocado, salt, pepper and lime juice into a bowl and stir.

2. Toast the bread to the desired doneness.

3. Cook the eggs, sunny side up.

4. Apply the mashed avocado on the bread slices. Place an egg on each slice. Sprinkle salt and pepper over the eggs and serve.

Double Berry Parfaits

Serves: 4

Ingredients:

- 4 cups plain Greek yogurt

- 2 pints fresh blueberries

- 3 cups sliced fresh strawberries

- The ground cinnamon, to sprinkle

- Honey to drizzle (optional)

Directions:

1. Take 4 Mason's jars or parfait glasses.

2. Add ¼ cup yogurt into each jar. Sprinkle some cinnamon.

3. Spread some strawberries followed by a layer of blueberries.

4. Repeat the layers (steps 2-3) until the ingredients are used.

5. Drizzle honey if using. Sprinkle cinnamon on top and serve.

Warm Fruit Bowl

Serves: 3

Ingredients:

- 1 cup blueberries

- ½ cup raspberries

- ½ cup blackberries

- ¼ cup chopped, fresh fig

- 2 tablespoons dried mulberries

- ½ ounce dark chocolate shaved

- ½ cup almond milk or oat milk or any other milk of your choice

- The ground cinnamon, to garnish

Directions:

1. Line a baking sheet with parchment paper. Spread the fruits on the baking sheet.

2. Sprinkle salt and cinnamon over the fruits.

3. Bake in a preheated oven at 375 ° F for around 20 minutes.

4. Remove the baking sheet from the oven. Scatter chocolate shavings over the fruit. Sprinkle cinnamon. The chocolate will melt because of the hot fruits. Toss well.

5. Divide into bowls. Warm the milk slightly if desired. Add milk on top and serve.

Second: Healthy Snack Recipes

Artichoke Pesto Mini Pizzas

Serves: 6

Ingredients:

- 12 ounces precooked, ready – to – heat polenta, cut into 6 slices of ½ inch each

- 1 tablespoon basil pesto

- 2 artichoke hearts, thinly sliced

- Fresh basil or thyme, chopped, to garnish

- 2 tablespoons low- fat marinara sauce

- 1/8 medium roasted red bell pepper, thinly sliced

- 6 tablespoons shredded, low- fat mozzarella cheese or Italian cheese blend

Directions:

1. Place polenta slices on a baking sheet lined with parchment paper.

2. Bake in a preheated oven at 400° F until for about 16-18 minutes. Flip sides halfway through baking. Take out the baking sheet from the oven.

3. Spread a teaspoon of marinara sauce on each polenta slice followed by ½ teaspoon pesto.

4. Place bell pepper strips and artichoke slices. Sprinkle a tablespoon cheese on each.

5. Set the oven to broil mode.

6. Broil for 2-3 minutes.

7. Sprinkle basil or thyme on top and serve.

Healthy Berry Yogurt Smoothie

Serves: 1

Ingredients:

- 1 ½ cups fresh blackberries

- 1 ½ cups fresh blueberries

- 10.6 ounces plain Greek yogurt

- 2 bananas, sliced

- 2 cups vanilla soymilk

Directions:

1. Add all the ingredients into a blender and blend until smooth.

2. Pour into 2 glasses and serve with ice.

Devilled Chia Eggs

Serves: 3 (2 halves each)

Ingredients:

- 3 eggs, hard-boiled, peeled, halved lengthwise

- ½ teaspoon chopped parsley

- ½ tablespoon chia seeds

- 1 ½ tablespoons mayonnaise

- A large pinch ground mustard

- Salt to taste

- Paprika to garnish

Directions:

1. Carefully remove the yolks from the egg halves and place them in a bowl. Mash with a fork. Set aside the whites.

2. Add mayonnaise, parsley, chia seeds, mustard, and salt into the bowl of yolks and mix well.

3. Fill this mixture in the cavity of the egg whites.

4. Sprinkle paprika on top. Chill for an hour and serve.

Frozen Peanut Butter Bites

Serves: 10

Ingredients:

- 1 cup crunchy peanut butter

- 1 over-ripe banana, chopped

- 1 scoop chocolate whey protein powder

- 1 tablespoon whole flaxseeds

Directions:

1. Add all the ingredients into a bowl and mix well using a fork until well combined.

2. Divide the mixture into 10 equal portions and shape into balls.

3. Place on a tray. Freeze until firm.

4. Transfer into a freezer-safe container and freeze until use.

Eggplant Parmesan Chips

Serves: 2

Ingredients:

- 1 small eggplant, cut into very thin, round slices

- 2 tablespoons freshly grated parmesan

- ½ teaspoon garlic powder

- Salt to taste

- Pepper to taste

- 1 tablespoon extra-virgin olive oil

- ½ teaspoon Italian seasoning

- Marinara sauce, to dip

Directions:

1. Place the eggplant slices on layers of paper towels. Sprinkle a little salt on it. Let it drain out some moisture from the eggplant slices for about 10 minutes.

2. Flip sides and sprinkle a little salt. Let it drain out the moisture for about 10 minutes.

3. Place eggplant slices in a bowl and drizzle oil over it. Sprinkle spices and Parmesan cheese and toss well.

4. Place the eggplant slices on a lined baking sheet, in a single layer.

5. Bake in a preheated oven at 350° F until for about 16-18 minutes.

6. Remove from the oven and cool completely.

7. Serve with marinara sauce.

Carrot Apple Muffins

Serves: 24

Ingredients:

- 3 flax eggs – procedure given in the directions

- 2/3 cup mashed, overripe bananas

- 1 cup unsweetened applesauce or finely grated apple

- ½ cup olive oil

- ½ cup agave nectar or maple syrup or honey

- 1 cup brown sugar

- 1 cup plain almond milk

- 2 heaping cups grated carrots

For dry ingredients:

- 1 teaspoon salt

- 1 teaspoon ground cinnamon

- 1 1/3 cups gluten-free oats

- 2 heaping cups gluten-free blend

- 3 teaspoons baking soda

- 1 cup almond meal

<u>To top:</u>

- ½ cup chopped or crushed walnuts

Directions:

1. To make flax eggs: For 1 flax egg, mix together 1-tablespoon ground flaxseed with 3 tablespoons water. Chill for 15 minutes. So make the flax eggs in this manner.

2. Grease 2 muffin tins of 12 counts each. Place disposable liners in it if desired.

3. Whisk together all the wet ingredients except carrots in a mixing bowl.

4. Stir in the carrots.

5. Add all the dry ingredients into a bowl and stir.

6. Add dry ingredients into the bowl of wet ingredients and stir until well incorporated.

7. Divide the batter into the prepared muffin tins.

8. Scatter walnuts on top. Press lightly to adhere.

9. Bake in a preheated oven at 375° F for 32 to 36 minutes until a toothpick when inserted in the center comes out clean.

10. Remove the muffin tins from the oven and place it on your countertop to cool. Remove the muffins from the tin and cool completely.

11. Serve. Leftovers can be stored in an airtight container in the refrigerator.

Zucchini Sushi

Serves: 4

Ingredients:

- 4 medium zucchinis

- 2 teaspoons sriracha hot sauce

- 2 cups lump crab meat

- 1 avocado, peeled, pitted, diced

- 2 teaspoons toasted sesame seeds

- 8 ounces cream cheese, softened

- 2 teaspoons lime juice

- 1 carrot, cut into thin matchsticks

- 1 cucumber, cut into thin matchsticks

- 1 cucumber, cut into thin matchsticks

Directions:

1. Make thin strips of the zucchini using a vegetable peeler. Place the slices on paper towels for a few minutes.

2. Add cream cheese, lime juice, and sriracha sauce into a bowl and stir.

3. Place sets of 2 zucchini slices (place one zucchini slice over another zucchini slice so make many sets like this using the zucchini strips).

4. Smear cream cheese mixture on the top slice of each zucchini set. Starting from one of the sides, place a little crab, carrots, avocado, and cucumber, next to each other. Start rolling from this side and place with its seam side facing down. You can also fasten with a toothpick.

5. Garnish with sesame seeds and serve.

Third: Healthy Lunch Recipes

Vegetarian Quesadilla with Broccoli Rabe

Serves: 2

Ingredients:

- ½ cup chopped broccoli rabe

- 2 whole-grain wheat tortillas

- ½ cup cooked or canned black beans, drained

- ¼ cup chopped onion

- 2 teaspoons olive oil

- ½ cup of corn

- ½ cup shredded cheddar cheese

Directions:

1. Place a pan over medium-low heat. Add 1-teaspoon oil and swirl the pan.

2. Scatter half of each – beans, onion, corn, broccoli rabe and cheese on one half of the tortilla.

3. Fold the other half over the filling. Cook until light golden brown. Flip sides and cook the other side until golden brown.

4. Make the other quesadilla similarly.

Zucchini Noodles

Serves: 4

Ingredients:

- 4 tablespoons olive oil
- 8 medium zucchinis, trimmed
- ½ teaspoon black pepper
- ¼ fresh dill, coarsely chopped
- 2 cloves garlic, minced
- ½ teaspoon black pepper
- ¼ cup chopped dill
- Fried or poached egg to serve (optional)

Directions:

1. Make noodles of the zucchini using a spiralizer or a julienne peeler.

2. Place a large skillet over medium heat. Add oil. When the oil is heated, add garlic and sauté for a few seconds until light brown.

3. Stir in the zucchini noodles. Add salt and pepper and toss well. Cook until slightly tender. Toss frequently.

4. Garnish with feta cheese and dill and serve.

Cobb Pizza

Serve: 2

Ingredients:

- 5 ounces refrigerated fresh whole wheat pizza dough

- 1 tablespoon low-fat buttermilk

- ¼ cup halved cherry tomatoes

- 1 ½ ounces boneless rotisserie chicken breast, shredded

- ½ teaspoon extra-virgin olive oil

- 1 bacon slice, cooked, crumbled

- 1 small ripe avocado, chopped

- 2 tablespoons 2% reduced-fat Greek yogurt

- 1 tablespoon canola mayonnaise

- 2 tablespoons sliced red onions

- ¾ ounce part-skim mozzarella cheese, shredded

- 2 tablespoons crumbled blue cheese

- ¼ cup packed arugula

- Pepper to taste

Directions:

1. Preheat a pizza stone or heavy baking sheet in an oven.

2. Thaw the pizza dough to room temperature.

3. Place the dough on a sheet of parchment paper. Roll the dough with a rolling pin and prick the dough at several places.

4. Lift the dough along with the parchment paper and place it on the preheated pizza stone or baking sheet.

5. Bake in a preheated oven at 500° F until for about 5 minutes or until light brown.

6. Add buttermilk, yogurt, and mayonnaise into a bowl and stir. Spoon it over the crust and spread it evenly. Do not spread around the edges.

7. Scatter tomatoes, chicken and onion over the crust. Sprinkle mozzarella on top.

8. Place it back in the oven and bake for 5 minutes.

9. Add arugula into a bowl. Drizzle oil over it. Top the pizza with this mixture.

10. Sprinkle bacon, blue cheese, pepper, salt and avocado on top.

11. Cut into 4 slices and serve.

Tuna and Chickpea Pita Sandwiches

Serves: 2

Ingredients:

<u>For dressing:</u>

- 3 tablespoons fat-free or low-fat Greek yogurt

- 4 teaspoons fresh lemon juice

- 1 teaspoon chopped fresh rosemary or ¼ teaspoon dried rosemary

- 2 tablespoons mayonnaise

- 2 tablespoons chopped fresh parsley

- ½ teaspoon chopped fresh thyme or 1/8 teaspoon dried thyme

<u>For tuna salad:</u>

- 1 can (4.5 – 5.5 ounces) white albacore tuna, drained

- 6 tablespoons chopped celery

- Salt to taste

- Freshly ground pepper to taste

- 1 cup shredded spinach

- ½ can (from a 15 ounces can) chickpeas, drained, rinsed

- 1 small red onion, finely chopped

- 1 medium tomato, sliced

- 1 whole-wheat pita pocket bread, halved

Directions:

1. Add Greek yogurt, lemon juice, rosemary, mayonnaise, parsley, and thyme into a bowl and whisk well.

2. Add tuna, celery, chickpeas, yogurt, salt, and pepper and fold gently.

3. Cut the pita halves thorough the center to make pockets.

4. Divide spinach and tomatoes among the pita pockets. Divide and fill the tuna mixture.

5. Serve.

Chicken and Brown Rice Soup

Serves: 4

Ingredients:

- 20 ounces ground chicken

- 4 tablespoons miso paste or soy sauce

- 2 cups spinach (optional)

- ½ cup lemon juice

- 6 cups water or chicken broth

- 4 cups cooked brown rice

- 3 tablespoons olive oil

- Salt to taste

- Pepper to taste

- Any other seasoning of your choice to taste (optional)

Directions

1. Place a soup pot over medium heat. Add oil. When the oil is heated, add chicken and cook until it is not pink anymore.

2. Add water or stock and rice and stir. When it begins to boil, lower the heat and simmer for 10-15 minutes.

3. Add miso paste, salt, pepper and lemon juice. Mix well.

4. Add spinach and stir. Turn off the heat.

5. Ladle into soup bowls and serve.

Tomato and Lentil Soup

Serves: 3

Ingredients:

- 1 tablespoon olive oil

- 1 stick celery, sliced

- 2 cloves garlic, peeled, finely chopped

- 6 tablespoons red lentils, rinsed

- 3 large ripe tomatoes, chopped

- 1 tablespoon milled chia seeds

- 1 carrot, chopped

- 1 medium onion, chopped

- 2 ½ cups vegetable stock

- 1 can (15 ounces) plum tomatoes

- ½ small bunch fresh basil, chopped

- Salt to taste

- Pepper to taste

Directions:

1. Place a soup pot over medium heat. Add oil. When the oil is heated, add carrots, onion, and celery and sauté until onions are translucent.

2. Add garlic and sauté for a few seconds until fragrant.

3. Add stock. When it begins to boil, add lentils and all the tomatoes. Let it cook for a couple of minutes.

4. Lower the heat and cover with a lid. Simmer until lentils are tender.

5. Turn off heat. Stir in the basil and chia seeds.

6. Blend with an immersion blender until smooth.

7. Add salt and pepper.

8. Ladle into soup bowls and serve.

Grilled Steak Tortilla Salad

Serves: 2

Ingredients:

- ¾ pound skirt steak

- Salt to taste

- ¾ pound plum tomatoes, chopped

- 1 small jalapeño, thinly sliced

- ½ bunch arugula, discard hard stems

- Flour tortillas, to serve

- ½ teaspoon chili powder

- Pepper to taste

- 1 scallion, sliced

- 1 tablespoon fresh lime juice

- ½ cup fresh cilantro

Directions:

1. Sprinkle chili powder, salt, and pepper over the steak.

2. Broil in a preheated oven for about 4 minutes. Flip sides and broil for another 4 minutes or cook to the desired doneness.

3. Place on your cutting board. When cool enough to handle, cut into slices.

4. Add rest of the ingredients except tortillas in a bowl and toss well. Add steak and toss again.

5. To char the tortillas: Place the tortillas directly on the flame for a few seconds until charred. Flip sides and char the other side as well.

6. Serve over charred tortillas.

Fourth: Healthy Dinner Recipes

Chicken and Sprouts Stir Fry

Serves: 2

Ingredients:

- ¾ pound chicken breasts, skinless, boneless

- 3 teaspoons olive oil, divided

- 1 clove garlic, peeled, minced

- 1 medium carrot, peeled, chopped

- 1 ½ tablespoon honey

- 1 cup bean sprouts, rinsed, dried

- ¾ teaspoon ginger, peeled, minced

- 2 scallions, chopped

- 2 tablespoons reduced-sodium soy sauce or to taste

- Salt to taste

- Pepper to taste

Directions:

1. Place a skillet or wok over medium-high heat. Add 1-½ teaspoons of oil. When the oil is heated, add sprouts and

stir-fry for a couple of minutes until light brown. Remove sprouts on to a plate. Set aside to keep warm.

2. Add 1-½ teaspoons of oil into the wok. When the oil is heated, stir in the chicken, carrots, garlic, and ginger and sauté for 2-3 minutes until chicken is light brown.

3. Stir in the scallions and cook until chicken is tender and brown all over. Stir frequently.

4. Stir in the soy sauce and honey and stir constantly for a minute. Turn off the heat.

5. Divide the sprouts among 2 serving plates. Divide the chicken and place over the sprouts and serve.

Korean Chicken Lettuce Wraps

Serves: 2 (3 lettuce wraps each serving)

Ingredients:

- 1 ¼ tablespoons soy sauce or to taste

- ¾ tablespoon dark sesame oil

- ½ tablespoon fresh, minced garlic

- ½ pound skinless, boneless chicken breast halves, thinly sliced

- 1 teaspoon canola oil

- 6 Bibb lettuce leaves

- 2 green onions, sliced on the diagonal

- 1 tablespoon dark brown sugar

- ½ tablespoon gochujang

- Pepper to taste

- ½ cup uncooked, long-grain brown rice

- ½ teaspoon toasted sesame seeds

- 12 English cucumber slices

Directions:

1. Add soy sauce, sugar, oil, gochujang sauce, garlic and pepper into a Ziploc bag. Seal the bag and shake until well combined.

2. Take out about a tablespoon of this mixture and place in a bowl.

3. Place chicken slices in the Ziploc bag. Seal the bag and turn it around to coat the chicken. Chill for 2-3 hours. Turn the bag around a couple of times during this time.

4. Follow the instructions on the package and cook the rice.

5. Place a skillet over medium-high heat. When the oil is heated, discard the marinade and place the chicken in the pan. Sear the chicken slices for 2-3 minutes on each side.

6. Turn off the heat. Add sesame seeds and stir.

7. Place the lettuce leaves on a serving platter. Divide the rice and chicken among the lettuce leaves.

8. Divide the green onions and cucumber slices among the leaves. Wrap and serve with retained soy sauce mixture.

Almond and Herb Crusted Baked Salmon with Asparagus

Serves: 2

Ingredients:

<u>For almond herb mixture:</u>

- 2 tablespoons ground almonds

- ½ tablespoon chopped fresh parsley or ¼ teaspoon dried parsley

- ½ tablespoon chopped fresh basil or ¼ teaspoon dried basil

- ½ teaspoon chopped fresh oregano or 1/8 teaspoon dried oregano

- Salt to taste

- Pepper to taste

<u>For salmon and asparagus:</u>

- ¼ pound small asparagus stalks

- 2 salmon fillets (6 ounces each)

- Zest of ¼ lemon, grated

- Juice of a lemon

- 4-5 thin lemon slices

- 1 teaspoon extra-virgin olive oil

- Salt to taste

Directions:

1. Mix together all the ingredients of herb mixture in a bowl and set aside.

2. Lay the asparagus on a large baking sheet. Pour oil over the asparagus. Sprinkle salt and half the zest. Toss and move the asparagus to one side of the baking sheet.

3. Place salmon on the center of the tray, with the skin side facing down. Drizzle lemon juice over the salmon.

4. Spread the herb mixture over the fish evenly. Sprinkle remaining zest over the salmon. Place lemon slices on top.

5. Bake in a preheated oven at 350° F for 12-15 minutes or until salmon is cooked through.

Grilled Halibut with Chia Pesto

Serves: 4

Ingredients:

<u>For chia pesto:</u>

- 2 tablespoons chia seeds

- 1 cup walnuts

- 4 large cloves garlic, peeled, smashed

- Salt to taste

- 1 ½ cups extra-virgin olive oil

- 6 tablespoons water

- ½ cup pine nuts or almonds

- 2 bunches fresh basil leaves (about 8 cups firmly packed basil)

- Freshly ground pepper to taste

<u>For halibut:</u>

- 2 tablespoons extra-virgin olive oil

- 4 halibut fillets (7 ounces each of about 1 inch thick)

Directions:

1. For the pesto: Add chia seeds and water into a bowl and set aside for 20-30 minutes to gel.

2. Transfer into the food processor bowl. Add walnuts, garlic, pine nuts, basil, salt, and pepper. Process until chopped into smaller pieces.

3. With the food processor running, pour oil in a thin stream. Process until smooth and well combined. Taste and add more salt and pepper if required.

4. Use as much as required in this recipe and transfer the remaining in an airtight container. Place in the refrigerator. It can last for 3-4 days. Use in some other recipe.

5. To make halibut: Brush oil over the halibut. Place on a preheated grill, with the skin side facing up. Cover the grill with the lid. Cook for 4 minutes. Flip sides and cook until fish flakes easily when pierced with a fork.

6. Remove fish from the grill and place them on a plate. Season with salt. Wrap the plate loosely with foil. Let it rest for 5 minutes.

7. Spoon a generous amount of pesto over the fish on top and serve.

Citrusy Shrimp-Stuffed Avocados

Serves: 2

Ingredients:

- ½ small shallot, finely chopped

- 1 ½ tablespoons sour cream

- 1 tablespoon orange juice

- ½ cup halved grape tomatoes

- 1 ripe avocado, halved, pitted

- Sweet potato chips, to serve

- 2 tablespoons mayonnaise

- 1 ½ tablespoon lime juice

- ½ pound cooked, shelled shrimp, chopped

- ½ Serrano chili, thinly sliced

- Salt to taste

- Handful cilantro, chopped, to garnish

Directions:

1. Add mayonnaise, shallot, lime juice, sour cream, salt, and orange juice into a bowl and stir.

2. Add shrimp, chili, and tomatoes into a bowl and toss. Add
   half the dressing and stir.

3. Fill the avocado halves with this mixture. Spoon remaining
   dressing on top.

4. Sprinkle cilantro on top.

5. Serve with sweet potato chips on the side.

Grilled Asparagus and Shiitake Tacos

Serves: 2

Ingredients:

- 1 ½ tablespoon canola oil

- ½ teaspoon ground chipotle chili

- 4 ounces shiitake mushrooms, discard the stems

- 4 corn tortillas, warmed

- 2 cloves garlic, crushed

- Salt to taste

- ½ bunch green onions, trimmed

- ½ cup guacamole

- Lime wedges, to serve

- Hot sauce, to serve

- Cilantro, chopped, to serve

Directions:

1. Preheat a grill to medium heat.

2. Add oil, salt, chipotle chili and garlic into a dish and stir.

3. Take out the asparagus and grill on the preheated grill until charred to the desired doneness.

4. Next place shiitake mushrooms and green onions and grill until charred to the desired doneness.

5. Chop asparagus and onion into 2-inch pieces. Cut the shiitake into slices.

6. Place tortillas on your countertop. Spread guacamole over it. Divide the asparagus, shiitake and green onions among the tortillas.

7. Garnish with cilantro, lime wedges, and hot sauce and serve.

Tuscan White Beans & Baby Kale

Serves: 6

Ingredients:

- 4 tablespoons extra-virgin olive oil

- 4 large cloves garlic, peeled, minced

- Salt to taste

- Red pepper flakes, to taste

- ½ cup chia seeds

- 1 teaspoon minced fresh rosemary or thyme

- ½ cup chopped, fresh, flat-leaf parsley

- 1 large red onion, diced

- 10 cups packed fresh baby kale

- Freshly ground pepper to taste

- 3 cups vegetable broth

- 2 teaspoons fresh lemon juice or white balsamic vinegar

- 2 cans (15 ounces each) cannellini beans or 3 cups cooked cannellini beans

Directions:

1. Place a nonstick Dutch oven over medium-high heat. Add oil. When the oil is heated, add onion and cook until translucent.

2. Stir in the garlic and cook for a few seconds until aromatic.

3. Add kale, spices, chia seeds, broth, and rosemary and lemon juice.

4. When it begins to boil, lower the heat and simmer until kale is cooked.

5. Stir in the beans and heat thoroughly.

6. Add parsley and stir. Taste and add more seasonings if required.

7. Serve hot.

Power Lasagna

Serves: 4

Ingredients:

- 4-5 whole wheat lasagna noodles

- 1 small zucchini, finely chopped

- 1 small green bell pepper, finely chopped

- 1 small onion, finely chopped

- ½ pound 90% lean ground beef

- 2 cloves garlic, minced

- ½ can (from a 14.5 ounces can) unsalted diced tomatoes, drained

- 1 tablespoon ground flaxseeds

- Pepper to taste

- Salt to taste

- ½ package (from a 10 ounces package) frozen spinach, thawed, squeezed of excess moisture

- 1 tablespoon white balsamic vinegar

- 2 tablespoons grated parmesan cheese

- ½ jar (from a 24 ounces jar) meatless pasta sauce

- ¼ cup loosely packed, chopped basil leaves

- 2 ½ teaspoons Italian seasoning

- ½ carton (from a 15 ounces carton) fat-free ricotta cheese

- 1 small egg, lightly beaten

- 1 cup shredded, part-skim mozzarella cheese

Directions:

1. Follow the directions on the package and cook the lasagna noodles. Set aside.

2. Place a skillet over medium heat. Add beef, onion, zucchini and bell pepper and sauté until the beef is not pink anymore.

3. Break the meat simultaneously as it cooks. Stir in the garlic and cook for a few seconds until fragrant. Drain off the fat remaining in the pot.

4. Add pasta sauce, basil, Italian seasoning, salt, pepper, tomatoes, and flaxseeds. Mix well. Turn off the heat.

5. Add ricotta cheese, egg, spinach and vinegar into a bowl and stir.

6. Take a square baking dish of about 8-9 inches. Spray some cooking spray all over the dish.

7. Spread ½ cup meat sauce on the bottom of the dish.

8. Place 2-2 ½ lasagna sheets in the dish. Spread 1-cup meat sauce.

9. Spread 10 tablespoons ricotta mixture over the meat sauce, followed by ½ cup mozzarella cheese.

10. Repeat the layers once more.

11. Finally, top with Parmesan cheese.

12. Cover the dish with foil.

13. Bake in a preheated oven at 350° F for about 20-25 minutes.

14. Uncover and continue baking until cheese melts and is brown at a few spots.

15. Remove from the oven and let it sit for 5 minutes.

16. Serve.

Conclusion

With that, we have come to the end of this book. I sincerely hope you found the book informative and the recipes easy to make.

As I mentioned before, the difference between a healthy and unhealthy life is just a matter of choice. It completely depends upon you if you want to choose to eat - healthy or not. Now that you have already taken the first step toward healthy eating for natural weight loss, it is time to put these recipes to use.

Make sure you focus on eating home-cooked meals. If you aren't able to cook every day, then you can try meal prep, which will give you access to tasty home-cooked meals any time you wish. You now have a list of ingredients through these recipes that you know are good for weight loss. You can use these ingredients to stir up your own recipes that are suitable for your taste buds and also convenient for you to prepare.

Thank you once again for choosing this book. I wish you luck in your journey toward a healthy life and natural weight loss.

Appendix A

Take the first progress photo

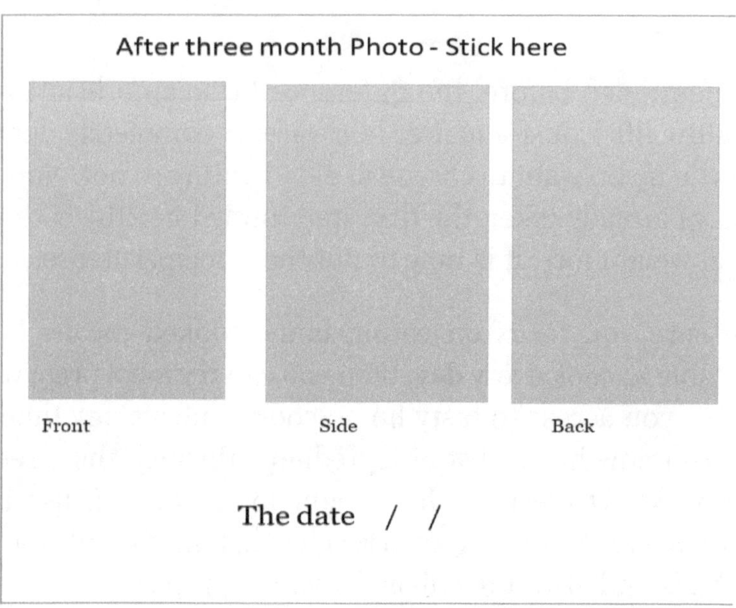

(Hint: a photo taken at the same distance, angle and lighting, wear tightfitting clothing to permanently reveal actual changes, keep the tightfitting cloth for more pictures)

Write several sentences to explain the states of your mood now:

Take the second progress photo

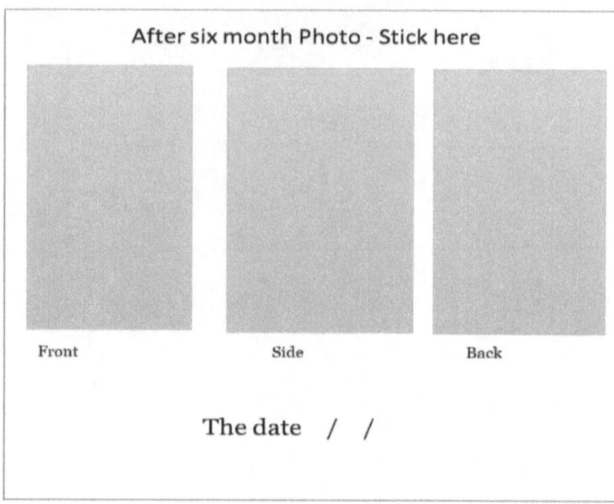

(Hint: a photo taken at the same distance, angle and lighting, wear tightfitting clothing to permanently reveal actual changes, keep the tightfitting cloth for more pictures)

Write several sentences to explain the states of your mood now:

Take the third progress photo

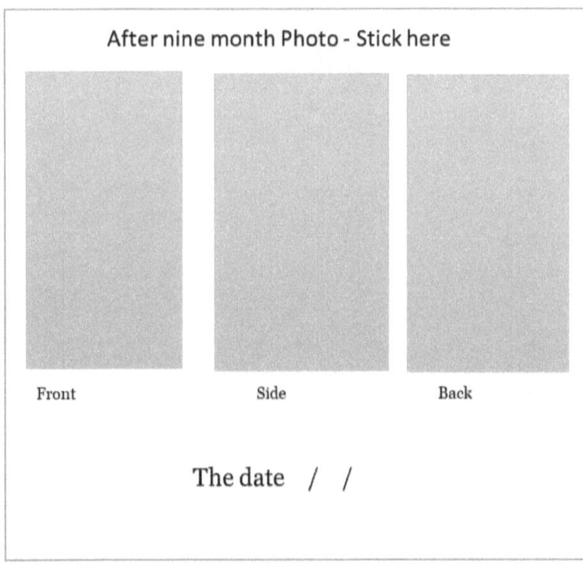

(Hint: a photo taken at the same distance, angle and lighting, wear tightfitting clothing to permanently reveal actual changes, keep the tightfitting cloth for more pictures)

Write several sentences to explain the states of your mood now:

Index

A

Accountability, 3, 16

Appendix A, 78

Avocado, 49

B

Baked Salmon, 69

Basic Rule, 3, 13, 16, 25

Berry, 50

Breakfast, 44

C

Carbohydrates and their benefits, 19

Cardio Training, 25

Chia, 46

Chicken, 64

Conclusion, 77

D

Dinners, 44

E

Eat, 1, 3, 6, 11, 16, 17, 18, 20, 36, 38

Every day, 44

F

Fats and their benefits, 20

Fitness method, 43

formula, 9

G

goals strategy, 31

Grilled, 66

Guidelines to Nutrition, 17

H

hungry, 41

L

Lasagna, 75

Lunch, 44

M

Meal preparation, 40

Metabolism, 3, 8, 9, 10

Move, 1, 3, 6, 11, 25

N

Noodles, 61

Nutrition, 38

O

Oatmeal, 47

P

Pizza, 62

progress photo, 79

progress schedule, 37

Proteins and their benefits, 19

Q

Quinoa, 45

R

recovery, 26

S

Scheduling, 3, 15

Shrimp, 72

Snacks, 44

Strength Training, 25

stuffed, 41

Supplement, 3, 23

T

Tacos, 73

The Road Map Plan, 28

Thermogenic, 23

Think, 1, 3, 6, 11, 13

Tomato, 65

Transformation, 27

transformation photo, 29

Tuna, 63

W

Whey Protein, 24

Workout, 42

Wraps, 5, 68

Z

Zucchini, 59